The Ultimate Hairstyle Handbook

Everyday Hairstyles for the Everyday Girl

by

Abby Smith

Second Edition

ACKNOWLEDGEMENT

This book would not have been possible without the kind support and help from my wonderful mother. No matter how crazy my aspirations, she's always believed in me and been my biggest supporter.

©2012, 2011 by Abby Smith
All rights reserved. First Edition 2011
Section Edition 2012
Printed in the United States of America
ISBN-13: 978-1481127165

I was a girl who hated my hair. It was dry, my ends were constantly breaking off and I couldn't grow it out to save my life. After heeding suggestions from my stylist, spending a few dollars on new product and lots of patience, I was finally able to grow long hair. And it was healthy and thick. Soft and shiny. Needless to say, I loved everything about it.

I wrote this book to share with you what I've learned over the last few years. I'm not a hairdresser, nor do I profess to be one. I'm just a girl with a passion for hair. I hope this book can provide you with a few extra tips on how to care for and style your hair.

<u>6 rules for long, healthy hair</u>

1) **Start out with healthy hair**. That's right. Chop off every inch of hair that is damaged. It's just non-negotiable. If you want healthy hair you need to start with healthy hair.

2) **Get it trimmed every 12-15 weeks**. Many stylists will tell you to trim your ends every six weeks. In fact, while I was growing out my hair that's exactly what I did. I trimmed it every six weeks and it took forever. I met a professional stylist from LA and he told me that it's unnecessary to trim your locks before twelve weeks.

3) **Do not wash your hair everyday**. Your best friend in growing out your hair will be the natural oil your body produces. It will strengthen your hair against the elements. It will keep it from drying out and breaking off. Wash your hair every 2-6 days to avoid stripping it of those natural oils. Did I just say 6 days? Sure did! I wash my hair once or twice a week. And no it doesn't stink, no it's not oily and yes I work out!

Two common complaints about rule number three: "Absolutely not! My hair gets way too greasy, there's no way I could go that long" and "I work out too much… I *have* to wash it everyday."

Here's the deal. Because you're washing your hair everyday—stripping it of those natural oils that we love so much—you're telling your body that it needs to produce more. You can't just wake up one morning and say, "Hey, I'm gonna go four days without washing you!" Because yes… that would be gross. **You've got to train your**

hair. Train it to do what you want. You are the boss. Go one extra day in between washings and give your hair time to acclimate to the change. When it stops producing as much oil, try going one more day! Give it some time though, your body needs it to get use to the changes.

Let me guess... you workout. And your hair gets so super wet around your face from sweating that you just *have* to wash it? Not anymore! Pull your hair up while you shower off and when you get out of the shower just blow the nape of your neck dry and where ever else it's wet. I promise it's not gross. Sweat is made up of mostly water. So just dry it and you'll never know the difference. If your hair is anything like mine you'll probably have a bunch of kinks in it when you get out of the shower. Immediately let your hair down after getting out the shower and brush it through while blowing it dry and the kinks should release themselves. Then just style it like normal.

If you must wash your hair every day, go easy on the straighteners and curling irons. Maybe even let it air dry one day. Avoid heat whenever possible.

4) **Spend money on products**. If you want to know what products I use, please refer to my products post at twistmepretty.com. The thing about products is they can be expensive… for cryin' out loud I'd rather buy a new pair of boots! But you need them. It's a love hate relationship really. The products I use have allowed my hair to not only grow long and healthy but stay long and healthy.

   1) Buy some thermal heat spray or serum. *I use Hana Shine from Misikko.* Please don't buy the cheap stuff! You usually get what you pay for. Depending on the serum, you can put it in while your hair is wet or you'll need to put it in after you blow it dry. I use a nickel sized amount and apply it to dry hair. You'll want to avoid putting the serum in your roots as it can cause your hair to look greasy if you use too much. If you're not washing your hair, use it before you use a straightener or curling iron. Whether or not I'm using heat, I use it everyday to tame frizz and condition my hair.
   2) If you have thin, lifeless hair you might want to try a volumizer/thickifier. *I use Small Talk by Bed Head.* I don't have super thin hair but there is a night and day difference when I don't use it. I use the product when my hair is wet, and because I only wash my hair every four to six days my bottle lasts forever.
   3) If you chemically treat your hair you should be using a product that has protein in it. *I use Anti-Snap by Redkin.* The protein will coat your hair, helping to defend it against the elements. I put mine in the ends of my hair when it's wet, making it another product that lasts.

4) Ever heard of dry shampoo? It's THE best product. You lightly spray it on your roots and it'll absorb the greasy oil and take away the unwanted sheen all while leaving in your natural oil to help strengthen and moisturize your hair. If you have thin, lifeless hair, or even short hair with choppy layers, you can use the dry shampoo to give your hair a great new texture. It also smells so yummy! *I buy the Suave Dry Shampoo from Walmart.*

5) **Avoid heat when possible**. I wash my hair, dry it and either curl or straighten it. The next day, if it's relatively straight or the curls are still in tact, I will wear it down again and maybe freshen up the pieces around my face. Day three I'll pull my hair half up, avoiding heat. By day four my hair feels dirty, so I pull it off my face into a bun, or side braid. If my bangs have gotten heavy and greasy, I'll wet them and dry them again helping them feel fresh and clean. Using dry shampoo can extend the life of my hair for another two days. The stuff is amazing. Avoid heat where you can.

6) **Take vitamins**. Hair is composed mostly of a protein called keratin. Multivitamins, prenatals or biotin can help assist the body in producing just that. Whichever you choose, always consult with a doctor first. The hardest part about taking vitamins isn't finding them… it's taking them consistently!

Tips and tricks

Don't wash your hair with super hot water. The heat from the water will suck all the moisture out of your scalp and open up your hair cuticle. Um… what does that mean? In a nutshell it means washing your hair in hot water can lead to dandruff and faded hair color. Watch out your hot shower takers! Right before you get out of the shower wet your hair down with cold water and it'll close the cuticle, leaving your hair feeling smooth. Rinsing with cold water will also lock in the color to help your color stay fresh and vibrant.

If you **swoop your bangs** like I do, blow them dry the opposite way you want them to lay. Then blow them to your normal side. Doing this will help your bangs swoop and it will also help keep your bangs from laying too flat on your forehead.

Use that little **nozzle attachment** your blow dryer comes with. It directs the hair cuticle downward giving you much smoother hair. When your hair is all dry, you can then remove the nozzle and mess up your hair just a bit.

Don't hairspray your hair until the end of the styling. When you spray your hair with hairspray before you curl or straighten it you are essentially baking alcohol into your hair. Yeah I know, that can't be good! If you need something to help hold curl, use a thermal spray or serum.

To help tackle frizz try not to roughen up your hair too much with a towel. Instead, work your way down the hair shaft or gently scrunch it. If you have curly hair try using a t-shirt instead of a towel. It's an old trick that helps eliminate frizz.

At the pool a lot? Before swimming please wet your hair down. If your hair has already soaked up some clean water it's not going to take in a whole bunch of chlorine. If you swim laps and use a cap, wet your hair down, condition it and then put your swim cap on. I was a swimmer in high school and it was the conditioner under the swim cap that saved my hair. Every day I got a good deep condition while my friends who didn't put conditioner under their cap were drying out their hair! If you like to lay out, apply a deep conditioner to your hair and put it up in a bun before you go. The heat from the sun will warm up the conditioner giving you a salon quality deep condition.

Keep the conditioner in your hair as long as possible. The second I get in the shower I shampoo my hair, rinse it and immediately put the conditioner in. That way the conditioner is working on my hair while I'm shaving and washing my body. You want to maximize the time the conditioner is in your hair. If you can, put your hair inside a shower cap and let the conditioner work on your hair for at least ten minutes.

Brush out the tangles while you are conditioning it. After letting the conditioner sit on your hair for a few minutes, brush out the tangles by using your fingers or a wide-toothed comb. Doing this will help evenly distribute the conditioner and make your hair that much easier to brush out when out of the shower. Harsh detangling can be traumatic, as your hair is most vulnerable when wet.

Ever gotten to that point when your **hair no longer wants to curl or straighten** for you? What you've done is removed all the moisture in your hair from the heat you've applied. Your hair needs that moisture to cooperate. Stop applying heat and please put some moisture back in it! Mist it with water or thermal spray, let it dry and come back to it.

Don't use grocery store bobby pins. They are not all created equal! If you want the hairstyles to hold, you must use strong bobby pins that stay closed. If you have thick, heavy hair, try using large bobby pins.

Need some volume? Use velcro rollers. First, mist hair with a styling spray. Then while your hair is warm from the blow dryer, wrap it up in some velcro rollers starting from the crown and working your way down. Warm your hair for a few minutes with your blow dryer, then freeze it out for another few minutes with the cold shot button. Finish getting ready and when you're all ready to go, take them out. It's like magic!

Try switching up your part. It will give those top pieces that commonly see all the heat, time to rest and cool underneath. You can also spray your paddle brush with some shine spray and brush your hair from mid shaft to ends. It will deposit enough product in your hair to calm the fly aways and frizz.

Clean your tools. Use some alcohol and a cotton pad to remove product residue. The old product can sear into your hair making it brittle... and we don't want that!

Remember to be patient. Whether your hair is not growing as quickly as you'd like, or you're having problems with some of the styles... keep at it! Your hair can be your best accessory if you treat it right.

This book comes with the password to many hairstyle videos that can be found on my website. The password to the private videos is **kangar00** (o's are zero's). Some videos are private and some are not. You can find my tutorials by going to the style gallery located underneath the hairstyles tab at the top of twistmepretty.com

xoxo Abby

Index of Styles

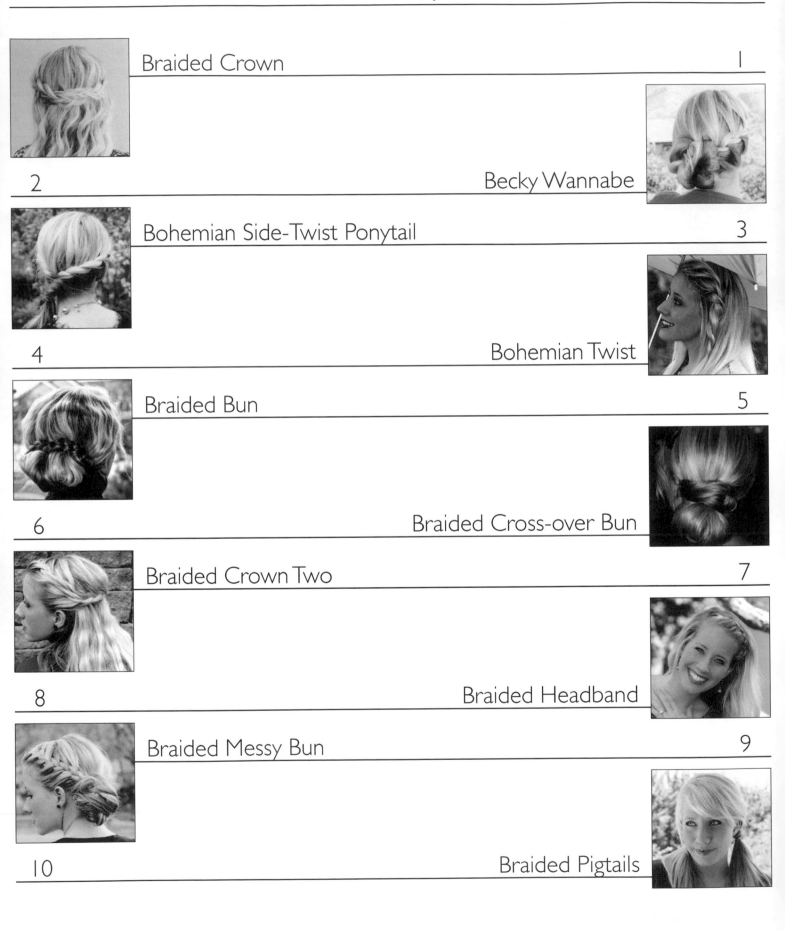

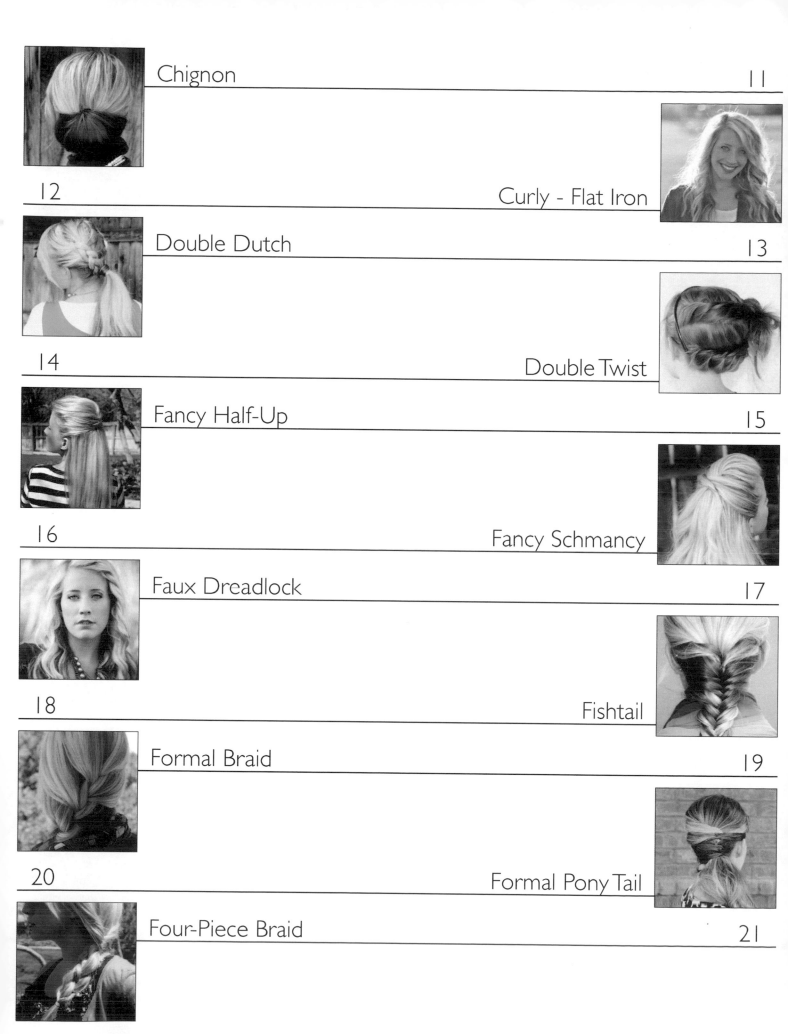

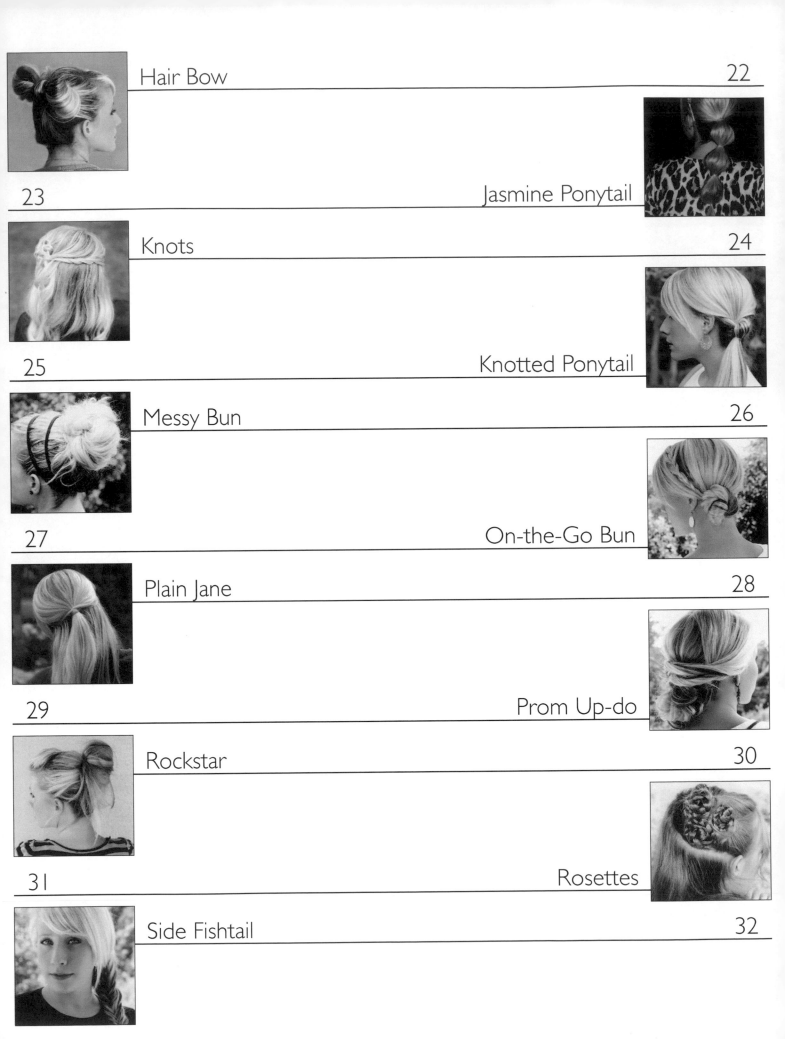

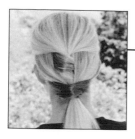 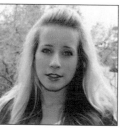
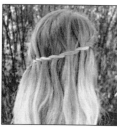
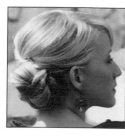

Braided crown

Note: Curl hair with wand

1. Gather front section of hair
2. Braid section
3. Tug and pull strands to loosen braid then tie off with clear elastic
4. Gather hair on opposite side
5. Braid hair
6. Tug and pull strands to loosen braid then tie off with clear elastic
7. Bring first braid back and around crown. Pin braid to crown of head
8. Bring second braid back and lay above first braid, making sure to hide tails. Secure with bobby pins

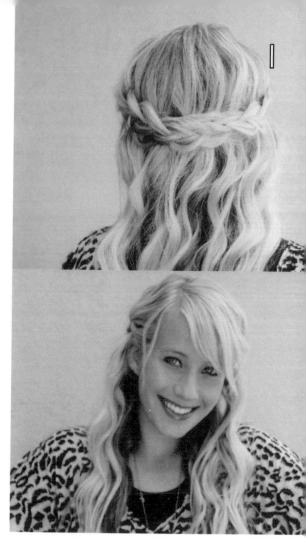

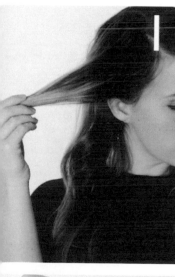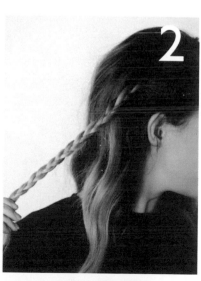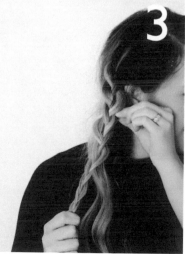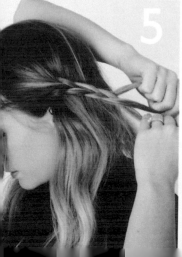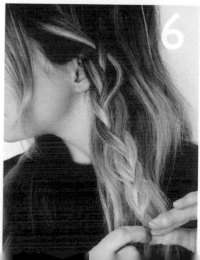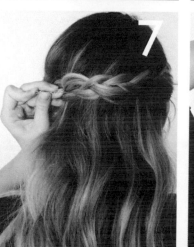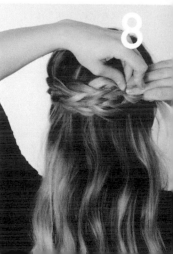

Becky Wannabe

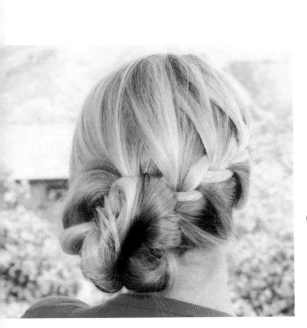

1-5. French braid hair across head

To french braid- Divide hair into 3 sections. Top section goes over middle section and bottom section goes over middle section. Then add hair to top section and braid over middle section. Add hair to bottom section and braid over middle section. Repeat

6. Either continue braiding and secure with elastic or tie tail into messy bun

Note: If braiding hair all the way down make sure to tug on sections of braid to make braid look fuller

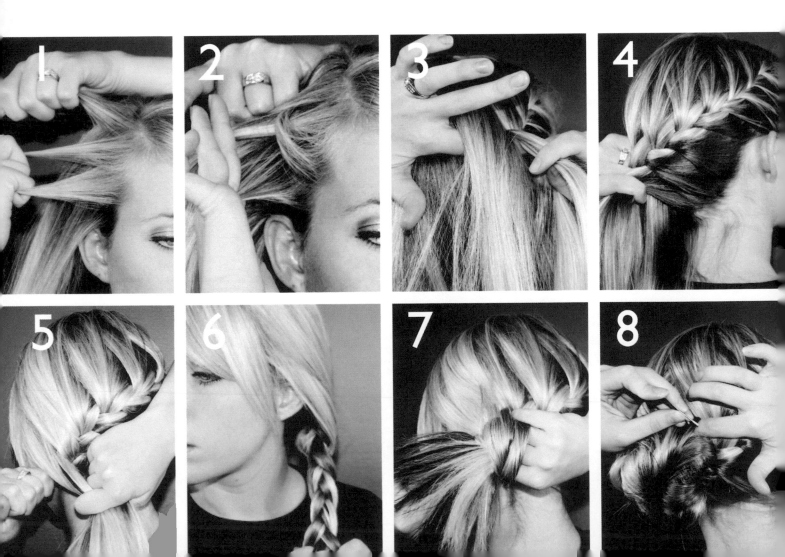

Bohemian Side-Twist Ponytail

1. Separate hair into two sections
2. Twist bottom section over top section
3. Add more hair to each section and twist bottom section over top section
4-6. Continue twisting around head
   Note: Refer to Bohemian Twist tutorial pg 4
7. Once twist reaches other side, secure with clear elastic
8. Just above elastic split hair and flip tail through hole

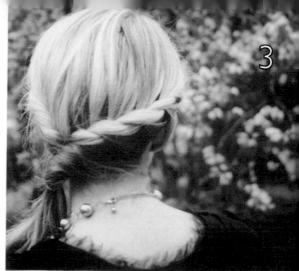

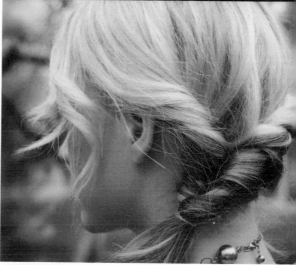

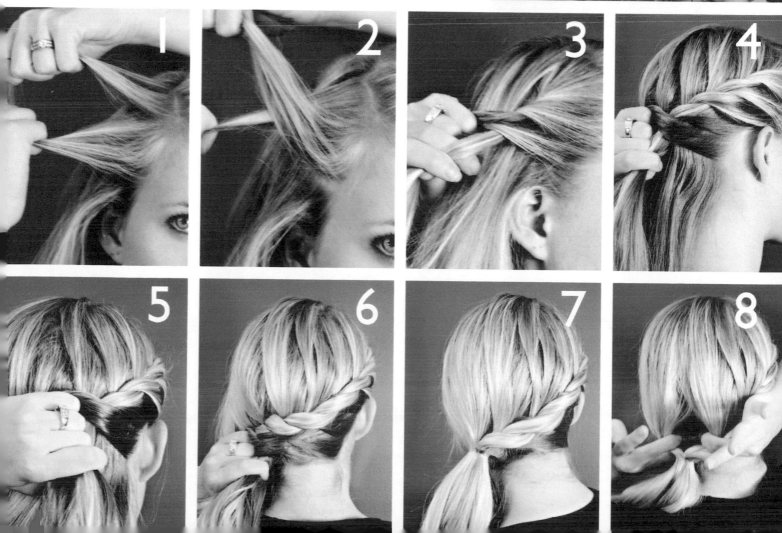

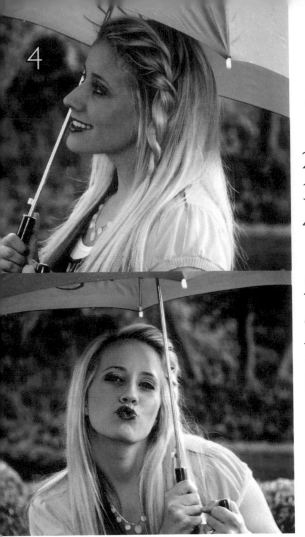

Bohemian Twist

1. Separate hair into two sections and twist bottom piece over top piece
2. Add hair to bottom piece
3. Add hair to top piece
4. Twist bottom piece over top piece
5. Repeat
6. Bobby pin hair in place
7. Continue twisting hair down
8. Secure with elastic band and hair will unravel making twist looser

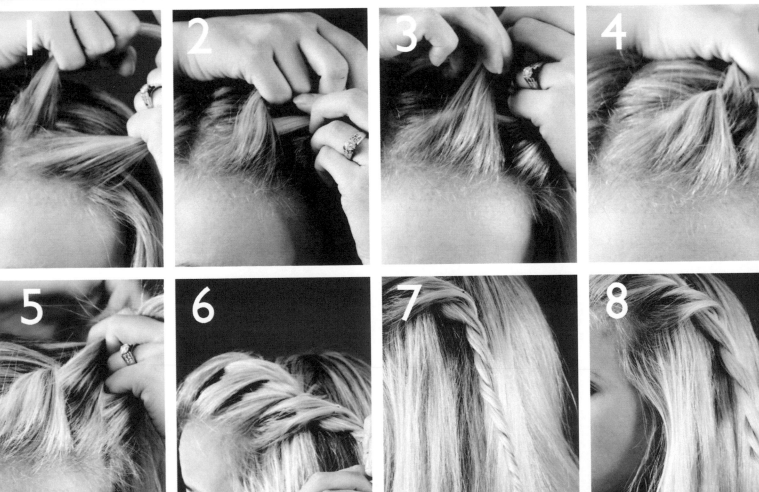

Braided Bun

1. Clip up hair leaving out two sections near nape of neck
2. Braid those two sections and tie off with clear elastics
3. Unclip and roll hair around finger
4-5. Secure hair using large bobby pins
6. Take right braid up and over rolled hair and secure with bobby pins
7. Take left braid up and over rolled hair
8. Secure with bobby pins and hairspray any flyaways

   Note: I slept in french braids to give my hair that three barrelled look

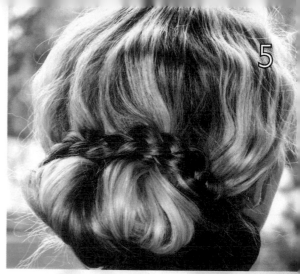

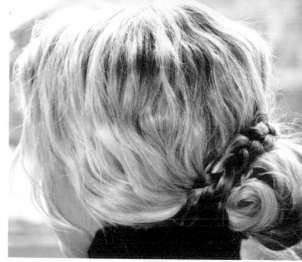

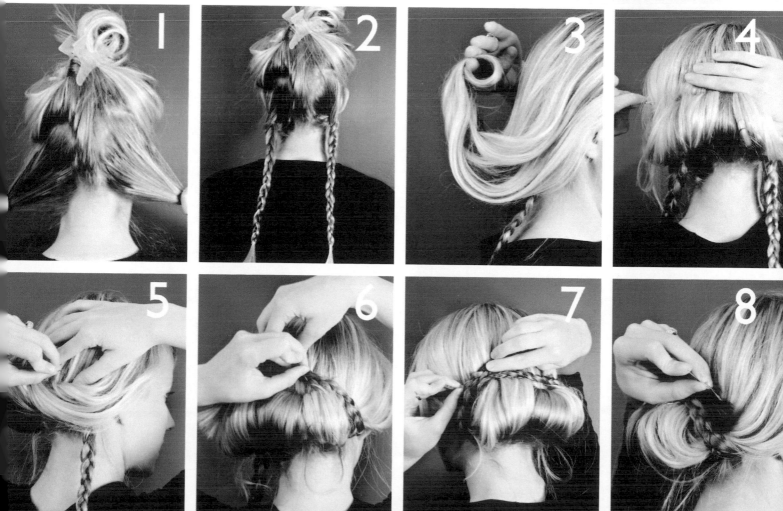

Braided cross-over Bun

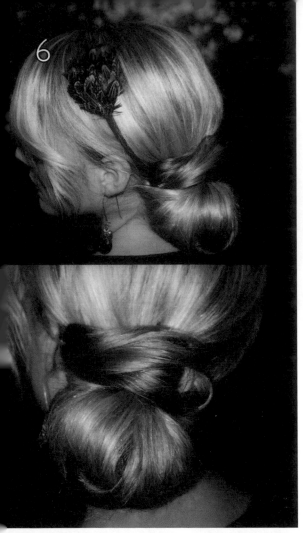

1-2. Make loose braid and roll around finger

3.   Secure into half bun with hair elastic

4.   Pull tail to tighten bun and to give you longer tails to cross over

5.   Take small piece of hair from left side and wrap loosely above braid

6.   Secure on right side with bobby pin

7.   Take small piece of hair from right side and wrap above braid

8.   Secure on left side with bobby pin. Continue wrapping until no hair left

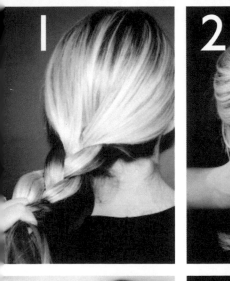
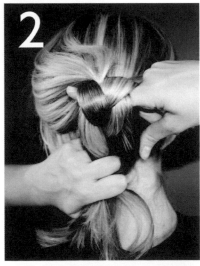
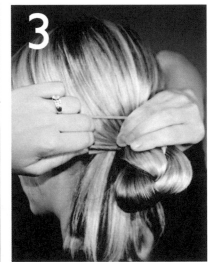
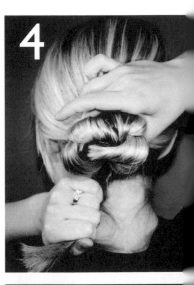

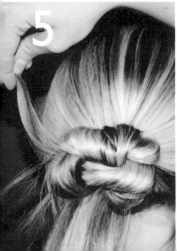
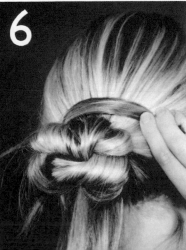
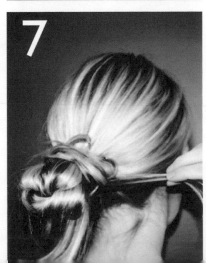
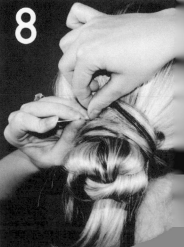

Braided crown Two

1. French braid bangs a few inches down head
2. Gather sections used in french braid
3. Divide gathered hair into 3 new sections to use in new french braid
4. Begin braiding hair across crown of head
5. Once you've reached the middle of head quit french braiding and continue a regular braid down the tail just in case braid loosens while you're pinning
6. Take bobby pins and secure it to head
7. French braid other side around head until it meets with other braid
8. Secure with bobby pins and three barrel rest of hair

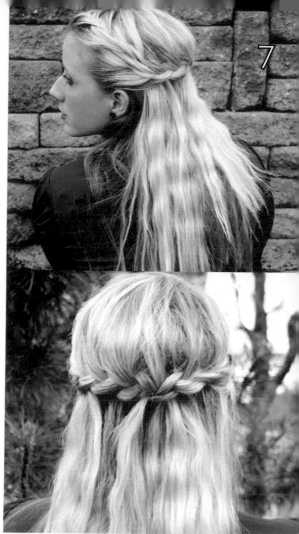

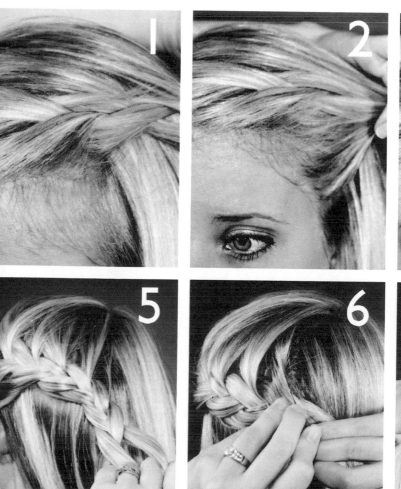

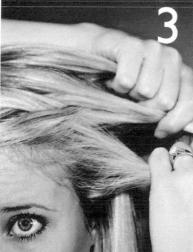

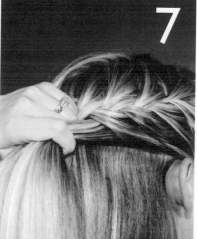

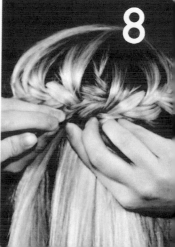

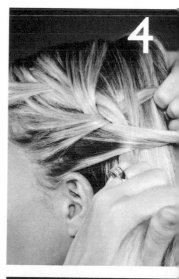

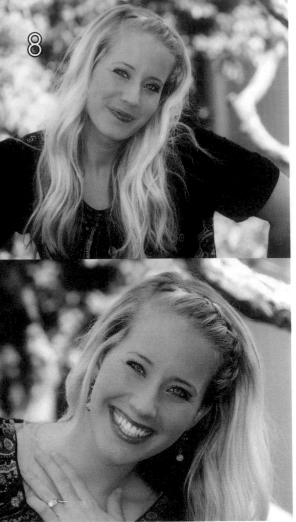

Braided Headband

1. Gather hair you want in headband using rat tail comb
2. Do two regular french braids down hairline
3. Continue with french braid only do not add piece of hair to top section of braid (one sided french braid). This will allow braid to pop up and be seen
4-5. Continue with one sided french braid all the way until top of ear
6. Secure hair with clear elastic band
7. Separate tail into two sections
8. Use a bobby pin to pin down tail closest to head. This will help tail to not poke out

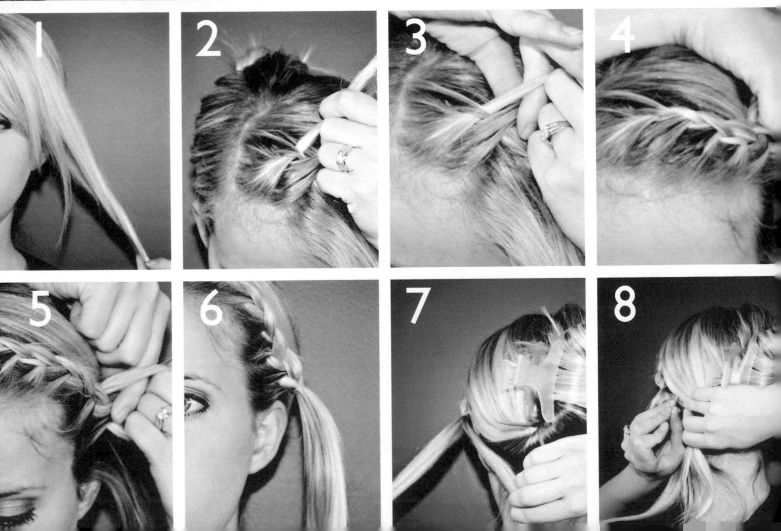

Braided Messy Bun

1-2. French braid hair down hairline. Stop at top of ear

3-4. Quit french braiding and braid tail. Secure at bottom with clear elastic

5. Rat side of head that is not in braid

6-8. Pull hair into a low side messy bun

Note: Refer to Messy Bun tutorial pg 26

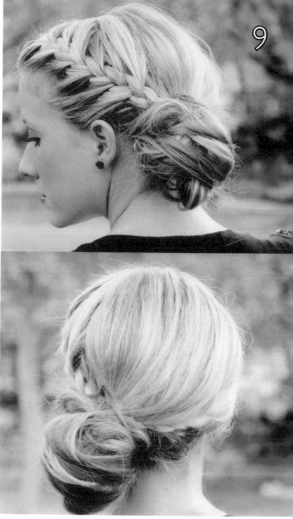

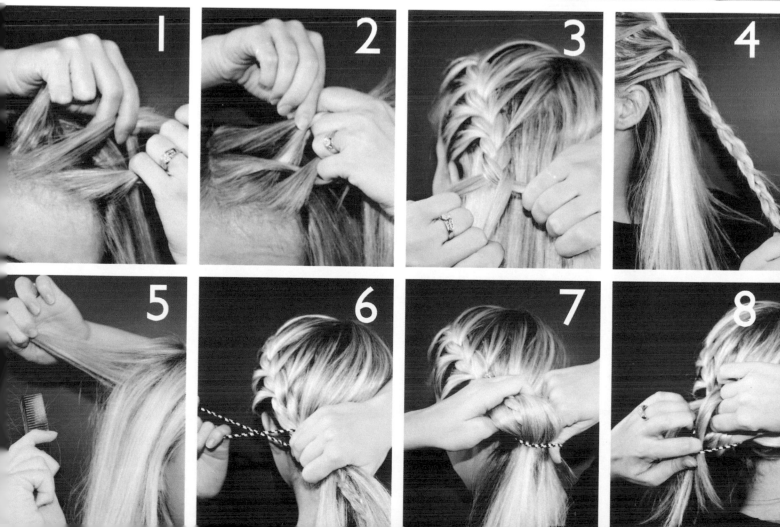

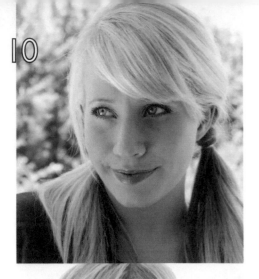

Braided Pigtails

1. Split hair down middle
2. Section off one side
3. Make loose french braid down back
4. Leave small piece out at nape of neck
5. Wrap piece around bottom of braid
6. Tie off braid with clear elastic
7. Repeat on other side
8. Tease tails to give them volume

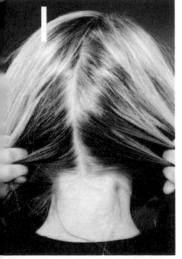

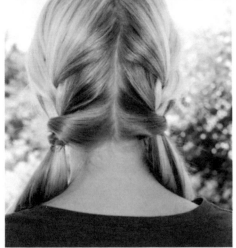

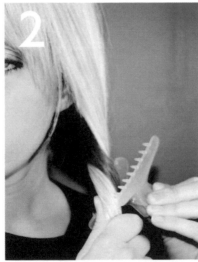

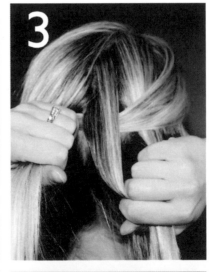

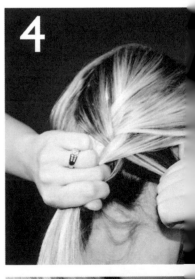

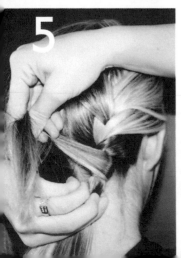

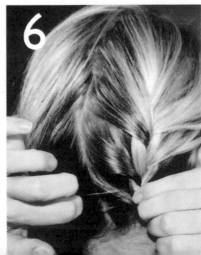

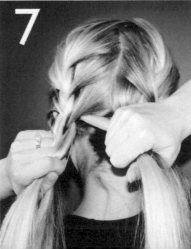

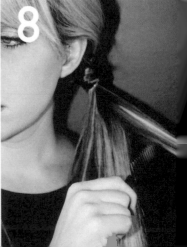

chignon

1-2. Rat hair

3. Pull hair back into low side half ponytail
   Note: Only take top layers of hair and make sure to leave a space in the middle for hair to go through

4. Rat tail

5. Tie off rest of hair with clear elastic. Make sure it's off center and that the tail is only a few inches long

6-7. Pull ponytail up and through hole

8. Tuck in ends and secure with bobby pins

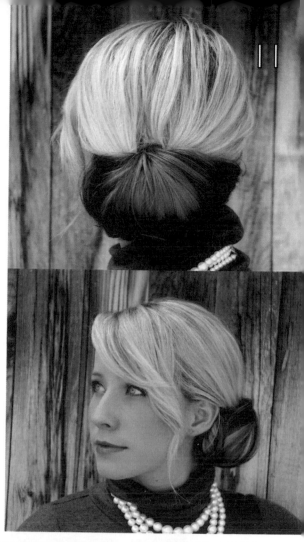

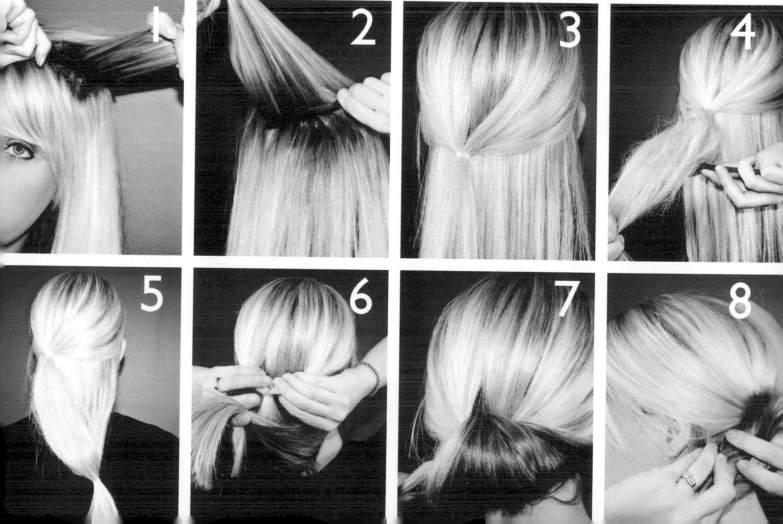

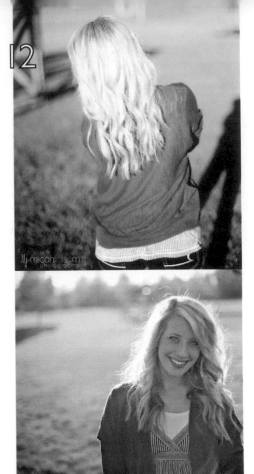

curly - Flat Iron

1. Section off hair from ears up
2. Start at the root of a section and begin curling
   Note: To curl, start with fingers forward on flat iron and rotate wrist so fingers end up closer to face. It's all in the wrist
3. Rotate wrist once and then pull straight down
4. When you get to the end, straighten the bottom inch to inch and a half of hair
5. Undo clip and take out more hair to curl

6-7. Repeat steps 1-5

8. Run fingers through hair and separate curls. Spray hair with hairspray while scrunching curls towards face

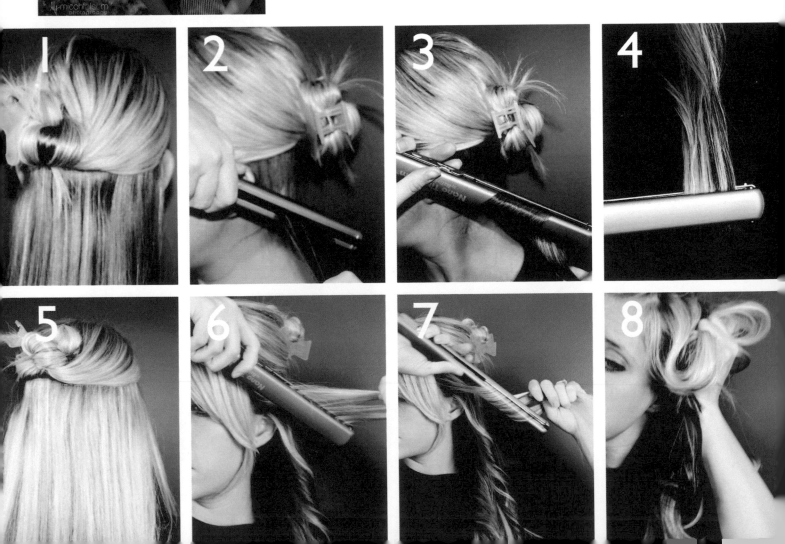

Double Dutch

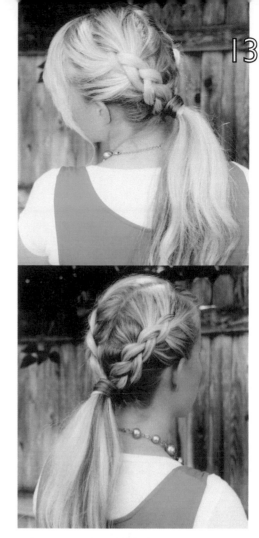

1. Divide hair into two sections. Section off one side with clip
2. Dutch french braid section of hair
   Note: Alternate crossing the two outer strands of hair UNDER the middle section instead of over as in a regular french braid
3. Tie off braid with a clear elastic
4. Dutch french braid other side of hair and secure with clear elastic
5. Combine two tails in middle and secure with clear elastic
6. Tug on braid to loosen and make hair look more full. Take out two clear elastics holding individual braids
7. Curl if needed and rat or tease the tail
8. Take a piece of hair from bottom of tail and wrap around clear elastic. Secure with bobby pin

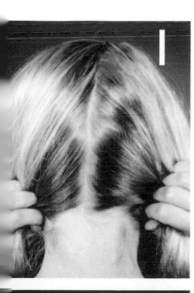

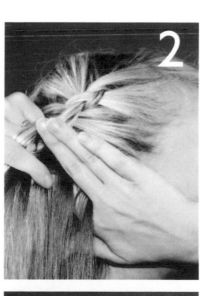

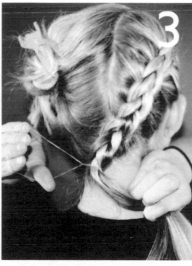

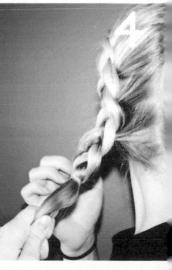

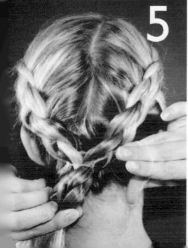

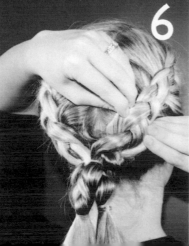

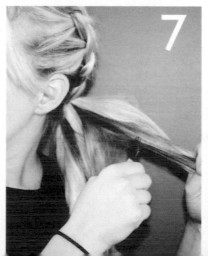

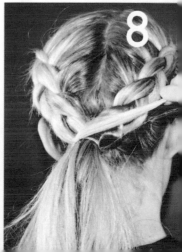

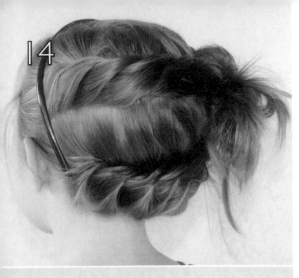

Double Twist

1. Split hair in half horizontally and secure top with clip
2-3. Bohemian twist bottom section across head
   Note: Refer to Bohemian Twist tutorial pg 4
4. Secure with clear elastic
5-6. Bohemian twist top section across head
7. Secure with clear elastic
8. Tie ends into messy bun and fix with bobby pins if necessary

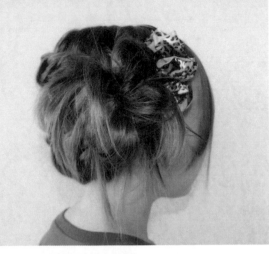

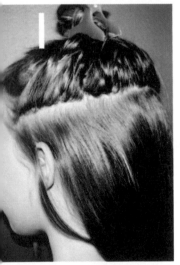

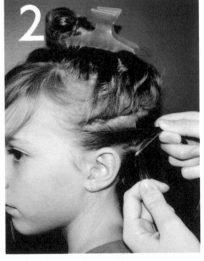

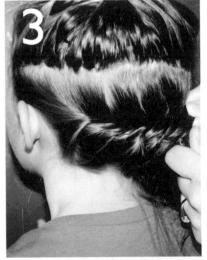

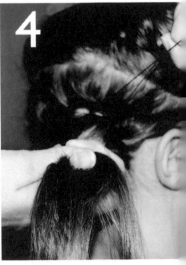

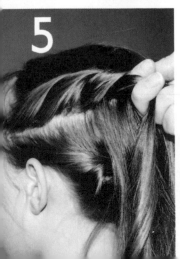

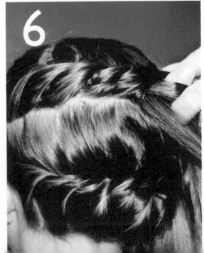

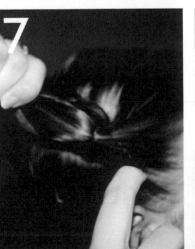

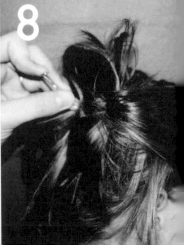

Fancy Half-Up

1-2. Rat hair

3-4. Pull hair back into half ponytail

Note: Do not pull all hair back. Only pull top layers of hair that show. This will help bobby pins hold hair better and will also make rest of hair look more full

5-7. Fold hair over itself

8. Secure with bobby pins

Note: Front layers of hair will hold back layers, so have bobby pins hold just those first few layers of hair

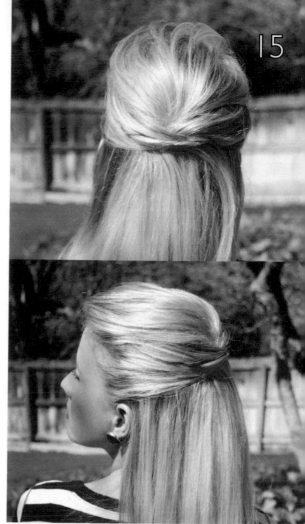

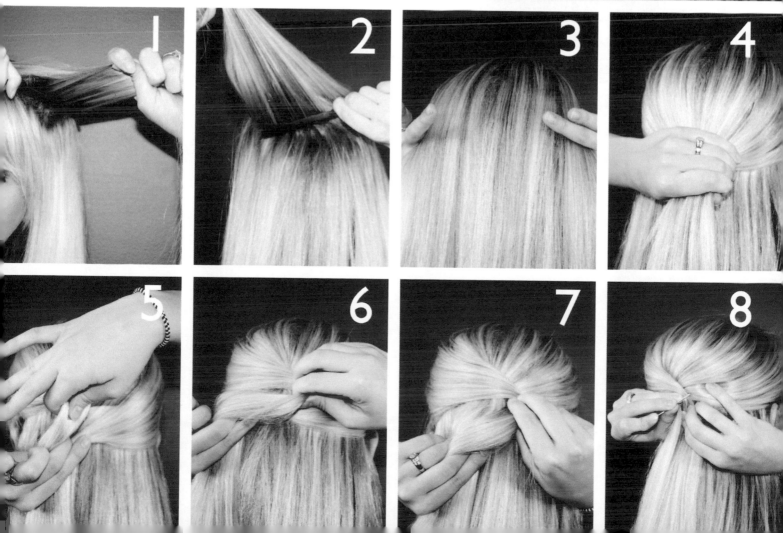

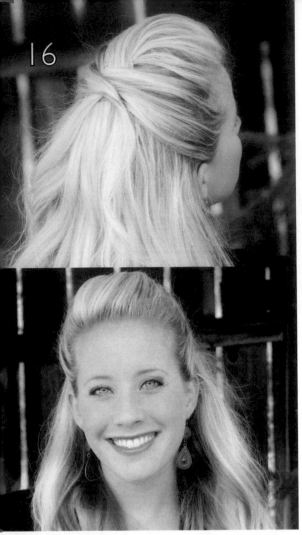

Fancy Schmancy

1-3. Pull bangs back and secure with bobby pin

Note: Do not let bangs lay flat on scalp. Tease hair if needed

4. Prepare another layer of hair for pinning

5. Take one side and pin it just below and to the side of first bobby pin

6. Bring other side over and secure it with bobby pin

Note: Make sure to cross sides

7-8. Repeat steps 4-6

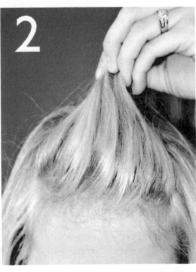

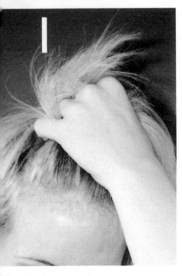

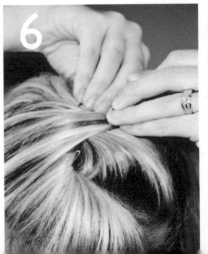

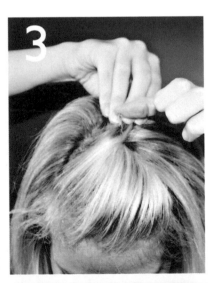

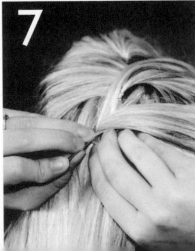

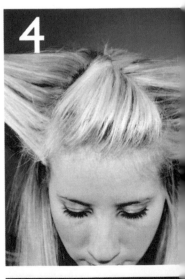

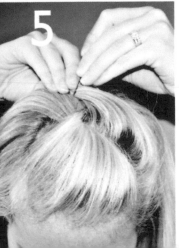

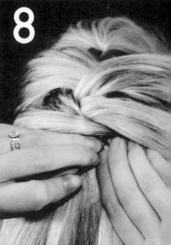

Faux Dreadlock

Note: Start with curly hair

1. Split hair into 2 sections
2. Twist up
3. Add a piece to the bottom section
4. Twist up
5. Repeat steps 3-4
6. Tie with clear elastic
7. Tug on twists, making them full and loose
8. Let go and twist will unravel

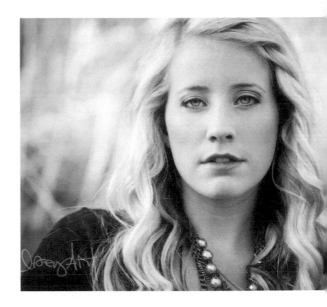

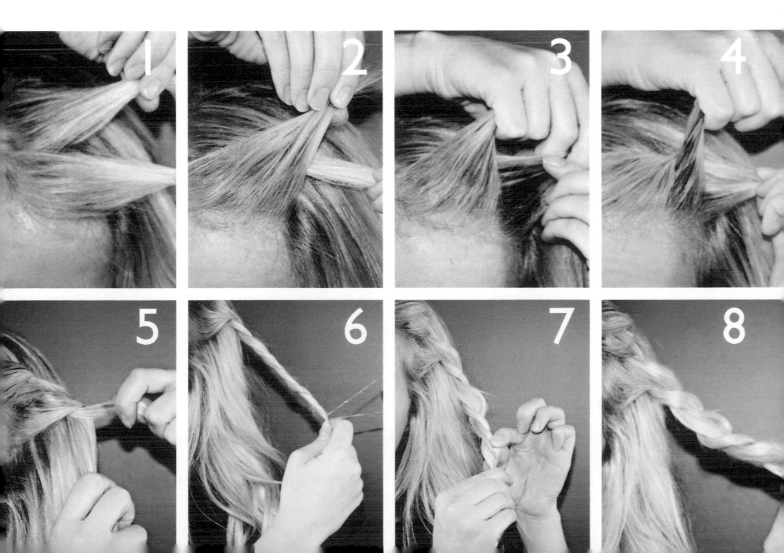

Fishtail

1. Pull hair up into half ponytail with clear elastic and split tail in half
2. Take thin section of hair from left side
3. Cross it over left piece
4. Combine it with right piece
5. Take thin section of hair from right side
6. Cross it over right piece
7. Combine it with left piece
8. Repeat until braid is finished

Note: To make it look fuller or messier tug on pieces of braid

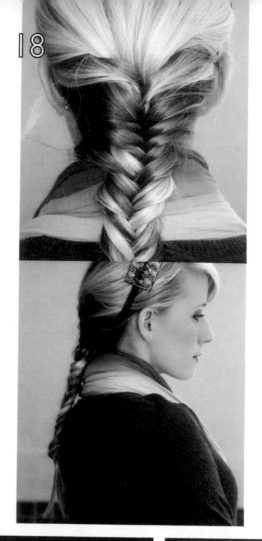

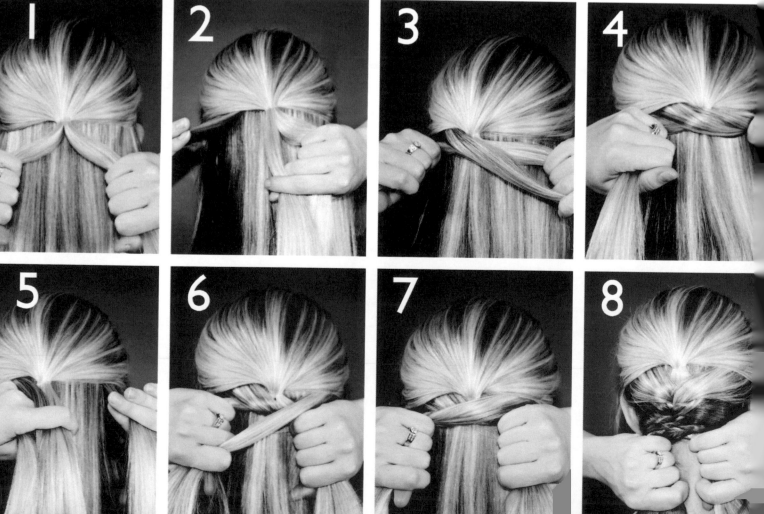

Formal Braid

1. Loosely pull section of hair from crown of head
2. Begin french braiding
   Note: Make braid loose and use large chunks
3-4. Continue braiding all the way down just past nape of neck
5. If needed, loosen hair and then secure braid with clear elastic
6. Loosen braid
7. Roll braid around finger
8. Secure roll with bobby pins

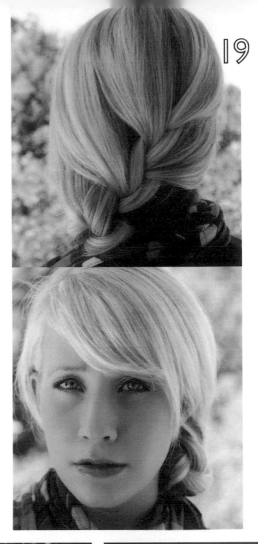

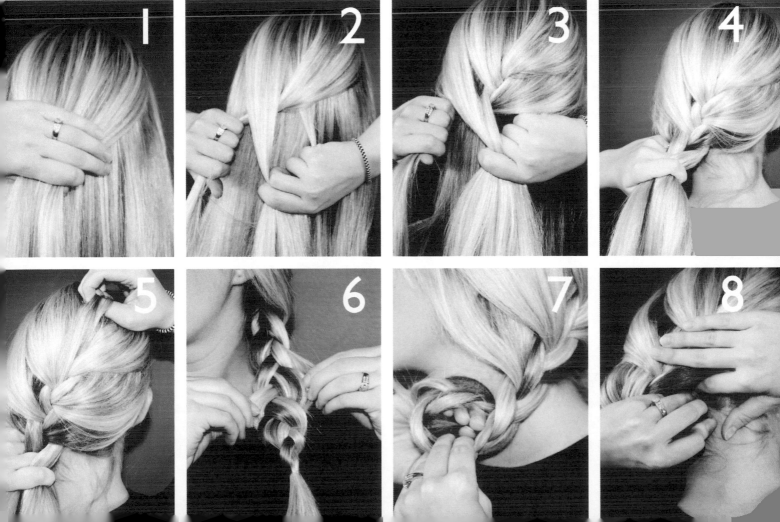

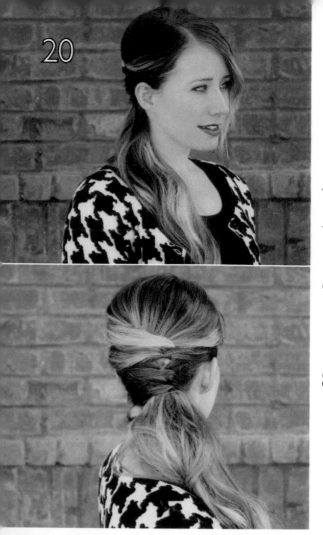

Formal Ponytail

Note: Start with curly hair

1-3. Bobby pin hair half up

Note: Refer to Fancy Half-Up pg 15

4. Take two thin sections of hair from front

5. Fold them over themselves and pin them directly below first bobby pin

6-7. Take two more thin sections of hair from front and pin them directly below first and second bobby pin

8. Take last sections of hair from bottom and pin directly below other bobby pins

Note: There should be a straight seam of bobby pins

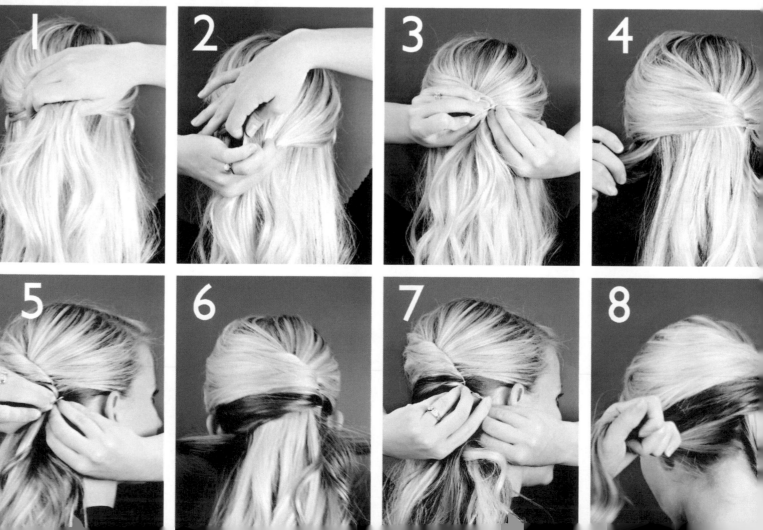

Four-Piece Braid

1. Divide hair into four sections
2. Piece 4 (furthest from face) goes over piece 3
3. Piece 4 goes under piece 2
4. Piece 4 goes over piece 1
5-7. Repeat

   Note: Always weave piece 4

8. Above braid, split hair into two sections and flip tail through hole just like a topsy tail

   Note: It will help if you do not look in a mirror and just concentrate on weaving. After a few passes you will see the braid start forming

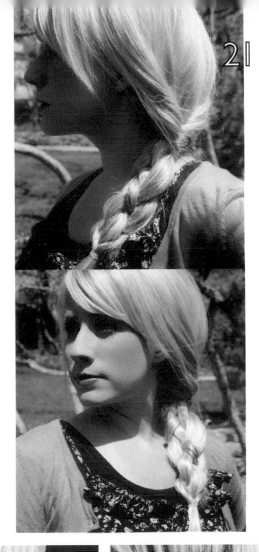

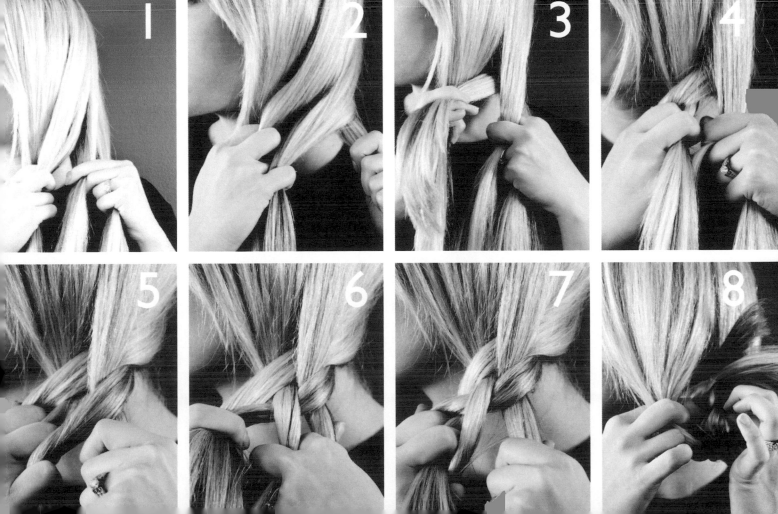

Hair Bow

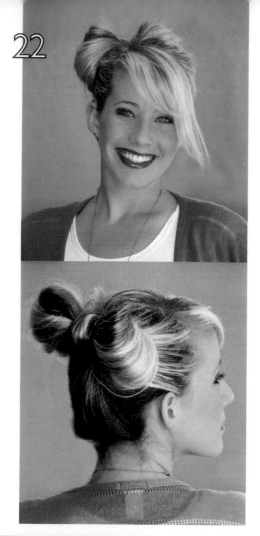

1. Pull hair into high half bun
2. Split bun into two sections
3. Wrap remaining tail forward
4. Secure tail with bobby pins
5. Bobby pin bow down
6. If necessary, spread bow to make bigger
7. Bobby pin bow down
8. Secure any pieces falling out onto sides of bow

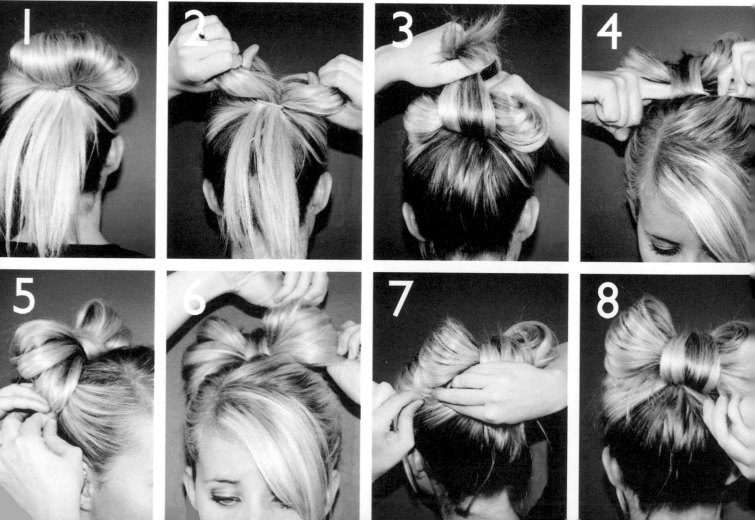

Jasmine Ponytail

1. Put hair up in ponytail
2. Rat tail
3. Add elastic 2 inches down from first elastic
4-5. Tug hair out of elastic to give it fuller bubble
6-8. Repeat

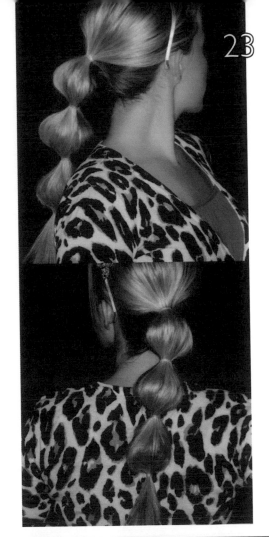

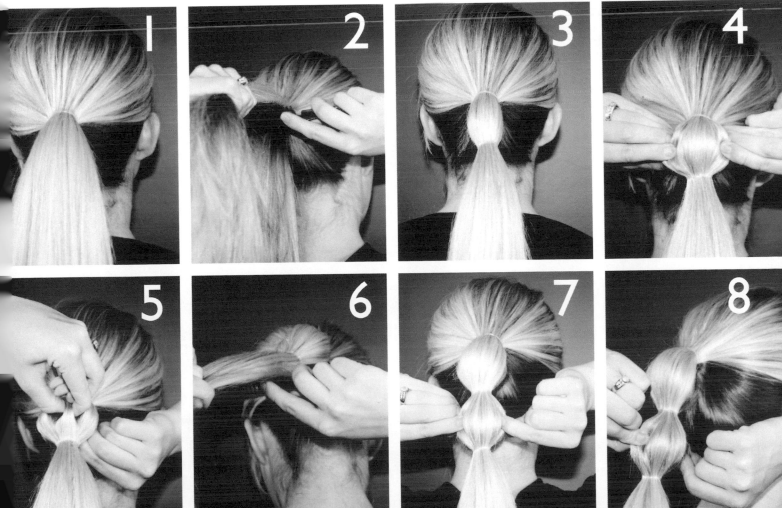

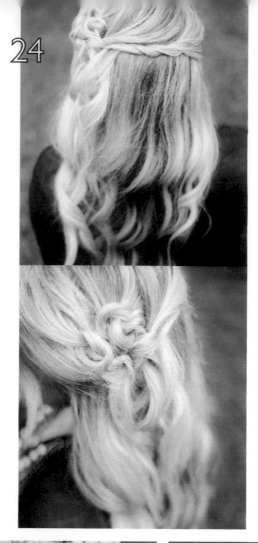

knots

Note: Start with curly hair

1. Take a chunk of hair from behind bangs, loosely tie in knot and bobby pin to head
2. Take another chunk, knot it and pin it to head
3-4. Continue adding and pinning knots until you've got a good cluster going on
5. Gather hair an inch above ear from the other side of head and pull it over to cluster of knots
6. Pin it
7. Take the rest of hair above ear and twist pieces together
8. Bring it over to cluster of knots and pin

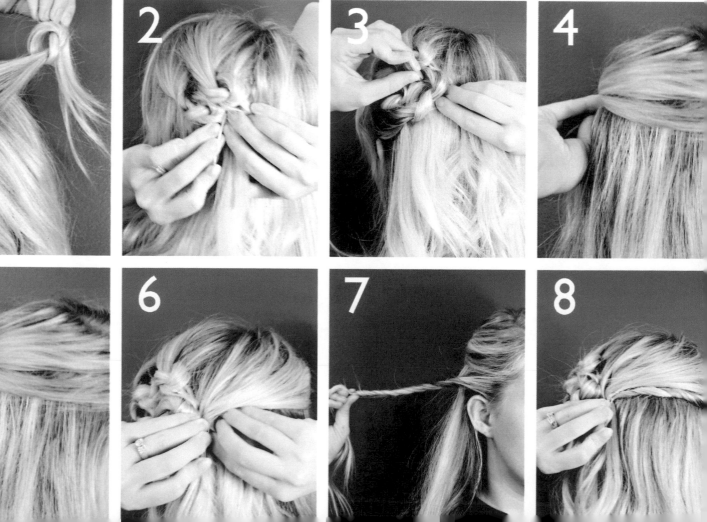

Knotted Ponytail

1. Pull hair half up and tie off with elastic band. Make sure it is sitting a little low and off center

2. Divide remaining hair into two sections

3. Knot those two sections around tail

4-5. Bring hands holding hair down and secure below knot with elastic

6. Break first elastic with fingers and push hair back into knot

7. Curl ends

8. Tease tail

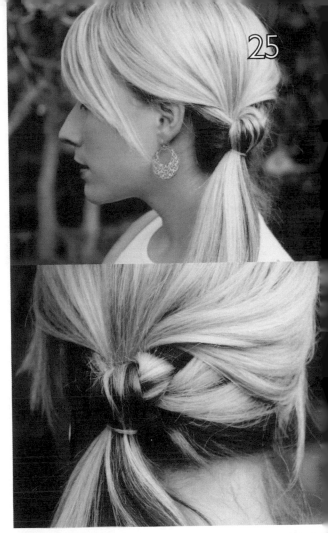

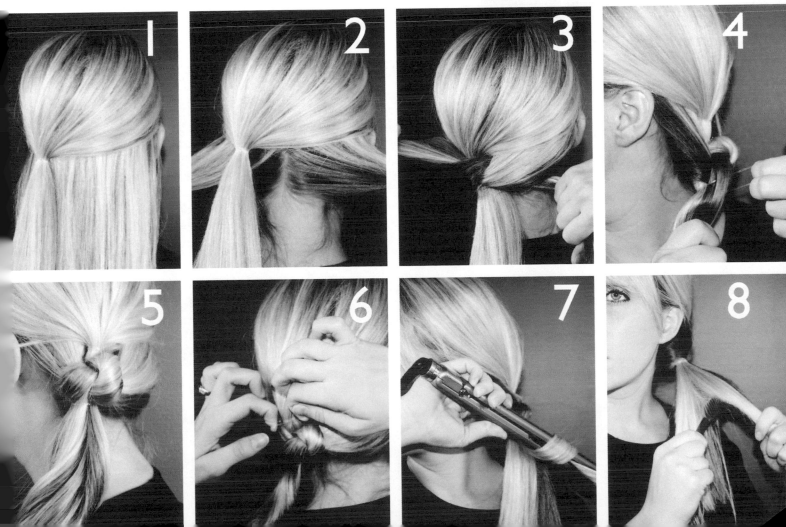

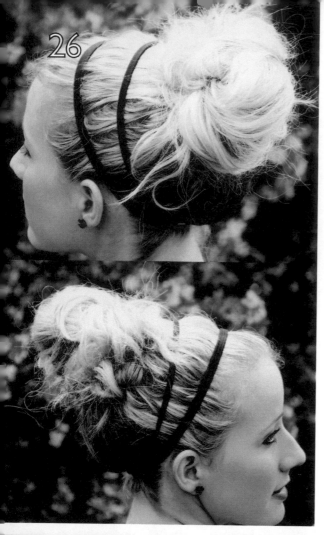

Messy Bun

1. Start with elastic on wrist. Pull hair through elastic
2. Pull hair through elastic again
3. Pull hair halfway
4. Twist hand underneath hair
5. Grab bun
6. Pull bun through elastic
7-8. Arrange and manipulate pieces by putting hair either back into elastic or bobby pinning them onto head

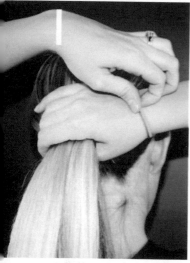
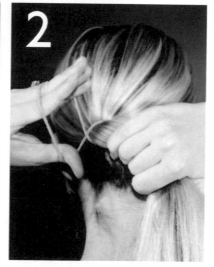
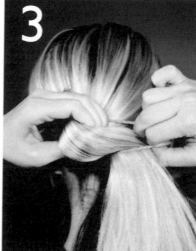
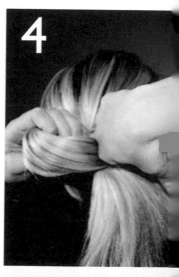
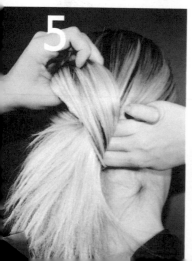
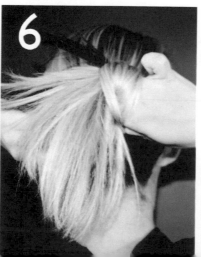
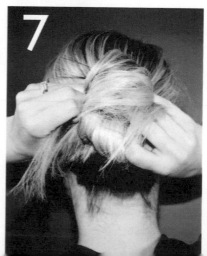
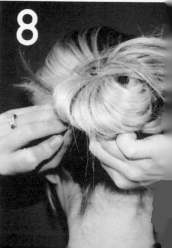

On-the-Go Bun

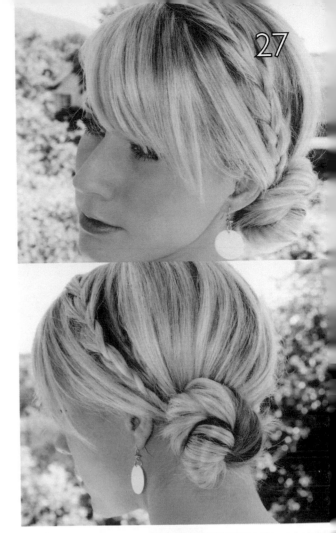

1. French braid small section of hair behind bangs. Once it starts falling, turn into regular braid and tie off
2-3. Braid a few more sections of hair
4. Tie off hair in low side ponytail
5. Twist hair
6. Start wrapping it into a bun
7-8. When bun is wrapped, secure with bobby pins

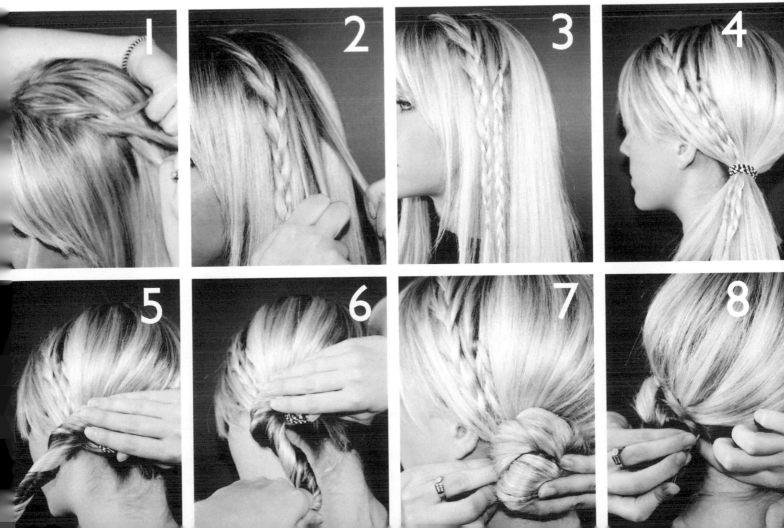

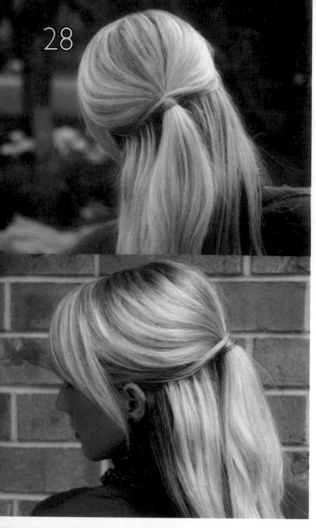

Plain Jane

1. Pull hair half up leaving out small sections in front
2. Take small section from one side
3. Wrap it around ponytail and secure with bobby pin
4. Take the other small section
5-6. Wrap it around ponytail and secure with bobby pin

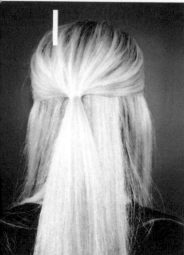

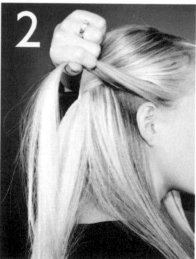

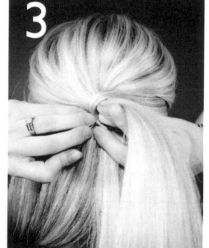

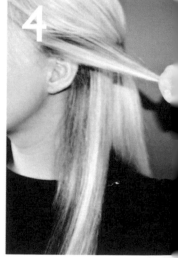

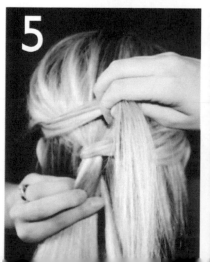

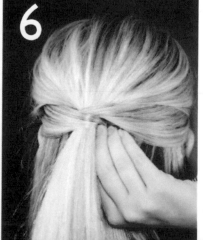

Prom Up-do

1. Start by sectioning off top layers of hair. Secure bottom layers in a messy bun
2. Twist small piece from top section and drape it over messy bun
3. Secure piece on opposite side with bobby pin
4. Twist small piece from other side and drape it over messy bun
5. Secure on opposite side with bobby pin
6-7. Repeat steps 2-5. Make sure to alternate pieces of hair

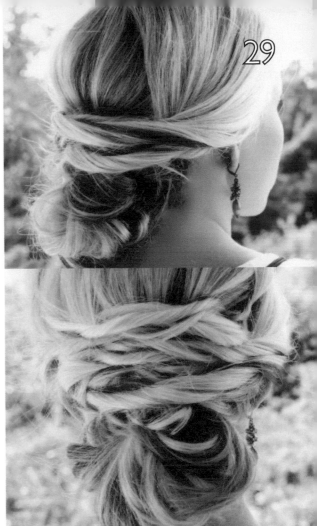

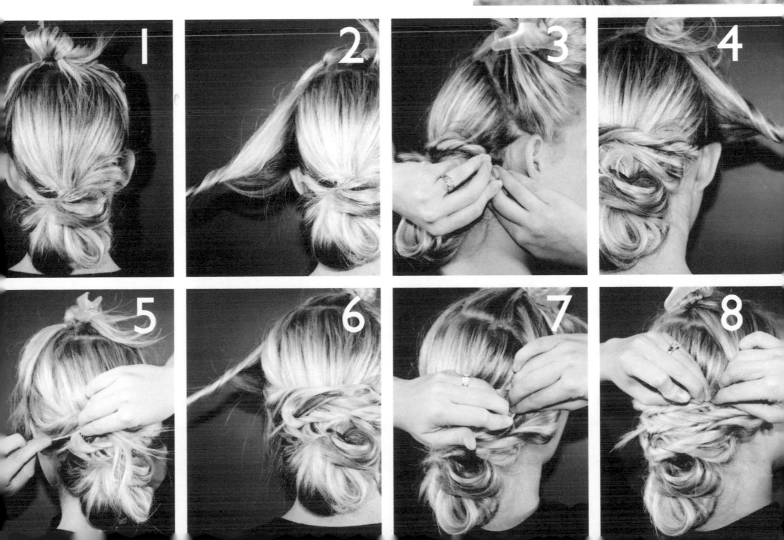

Rockstar

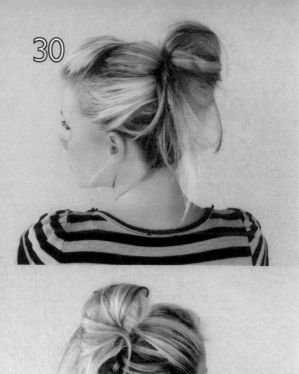

1. Pull bangs back with hand
2. While holding bangs, push them forward to create volume and secure with bobby pins
3. Pull up hair into high half ponytail and secure with clear elastic
4. Bend over, let rest of hair fall forward and begin braiding up (dutch or regular style)
5. Continue braiding until hair meets with first elastic
6. Flip over and secure with hair tie
7. Rat tail
8. Wrap hair into messy bun, secure with bobby pins if necessary

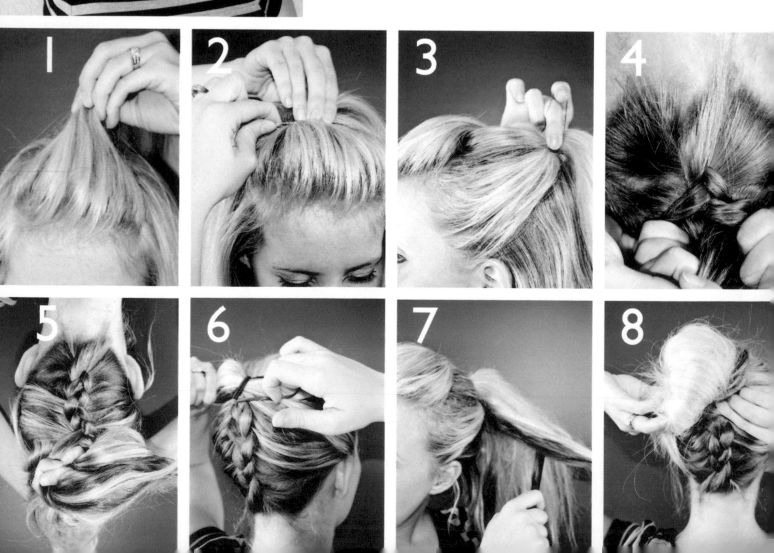

Rosettes

1. Section off hair
2. Split sectioned off hair in half horizontally, clip bottom hair and secure top half with clear elastic
3. Braid tail and roll into rosette
4. Divide bottom hair into two sections and secure with clear elastics
5. Braid tails and secure bottoms with clear elastics
6-7. Roll braids into rosettes, securing with bobby pins
8. Curl rest of hair

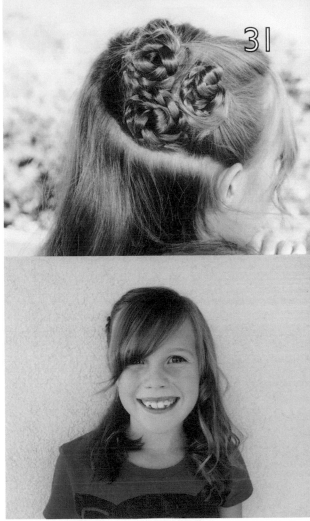

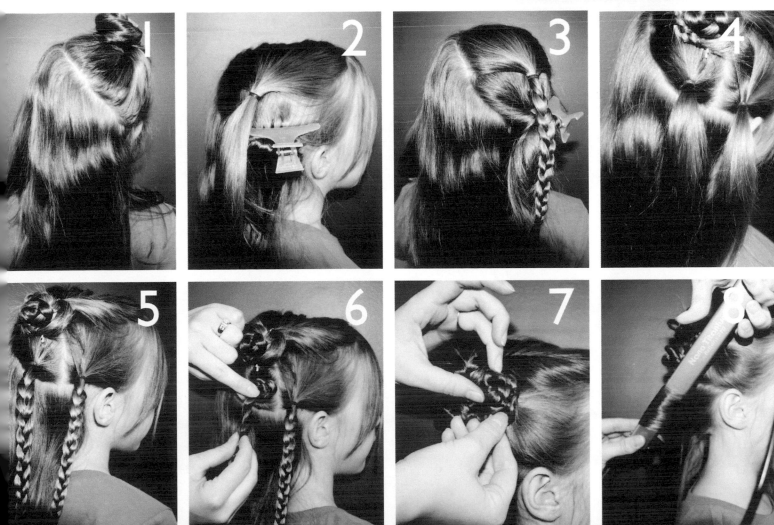

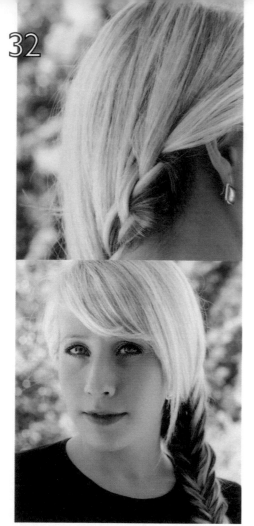

Side Fishtail

1-2. *Optional: Braid small section of hair from opposite side your fishtail will sit. Doing this will help shorter pieces stay in fishtail*

3. Split hair into two sections
4. Take thin section of hair from back of one of the sections
5. Wrap that piece forward and over the section it came from and combine it with other section
6. Take small piece of hair from the back of the other section
7. Wrap that piece forward and over the section it came from and combine it with other section. Repeat steps 3-7
8. Leave fishtail tight, or pull chunks out to make it look fuller and messier

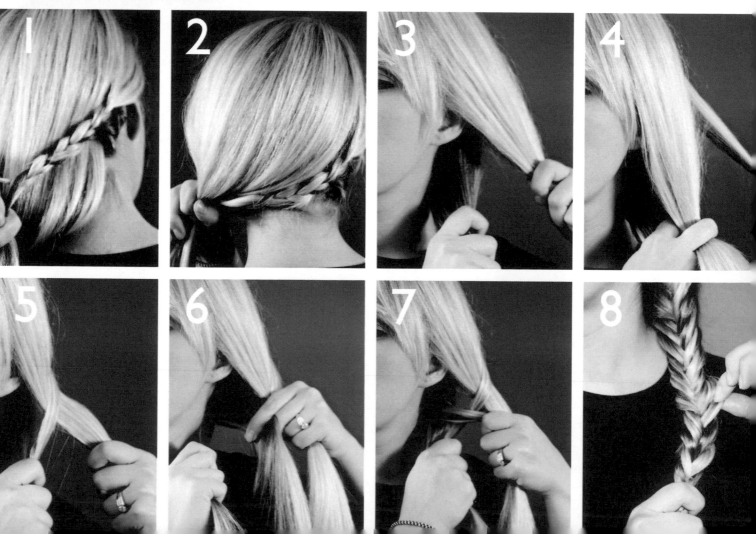

The Tennis Player

1. Pull hair half up and secure with clear elastic
2. Take a section of hair from below and wrap it around clear elastic
3. Bobby pin to head
4. Gather rest of hair into low ponytail and secure with clear elastic. Leave out a few sections near nape of neck
5. Take those two sections and twist around clear elastic
6. Secure with bobby pin

   Note: If you can see your bobby pin from the first wrap, take it out

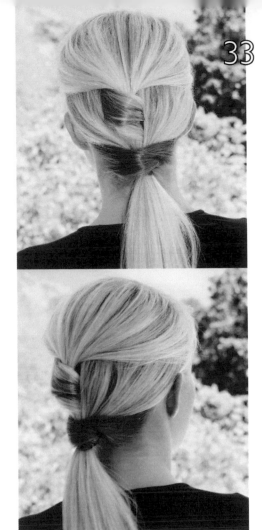

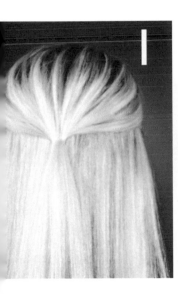

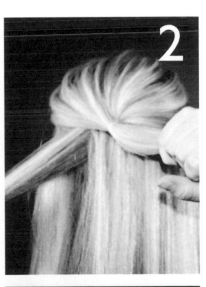

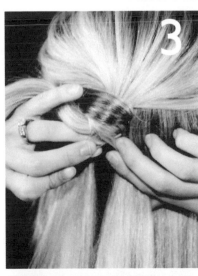

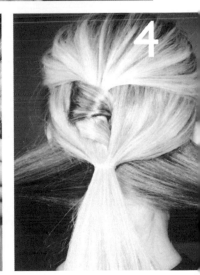

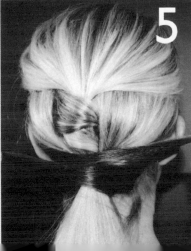

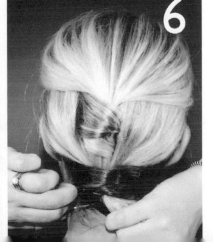

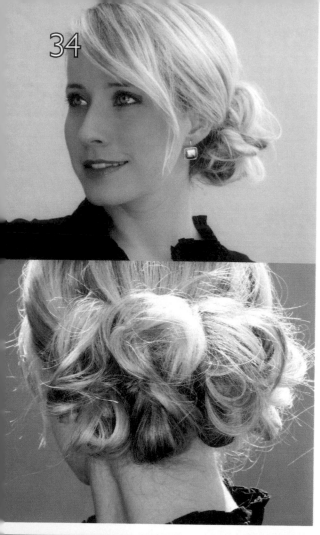

Three-Banded Buns

1-4. Take one third of hair and put into messy bun

5. If necessary, fix bun with bobby pins

6-7. Take middle section and repeat steps 2-5

8. Take last section and repeat steps 2-5

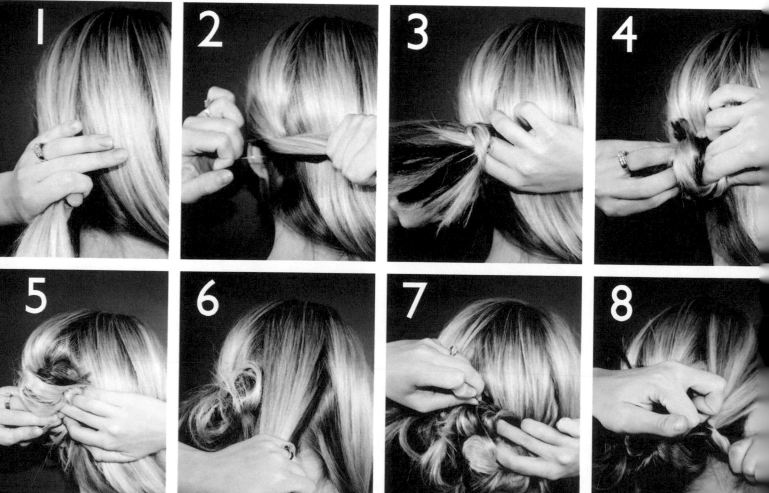

Throwback to the 30's

1. Pin bangs back
2. Roll section of hair behind bangs forward and pin
3. Sweep a chunk of hair back and pin it over step two's bobby pin
4. Sweep the rest of front section of hair back and pin it with step three's bobby pin
5. Pin a section of hair from opposite side into the cluster of bobby pins
6. Take tails of cluster, roll them into bun and pin
7. Tie top section of hair from opposite side into loose knot and pin
8. Tie rest of hair above ears into a knot and pin
   Note: Finish by curling the rest of hair

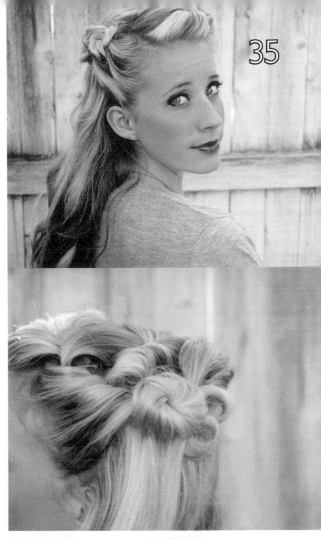

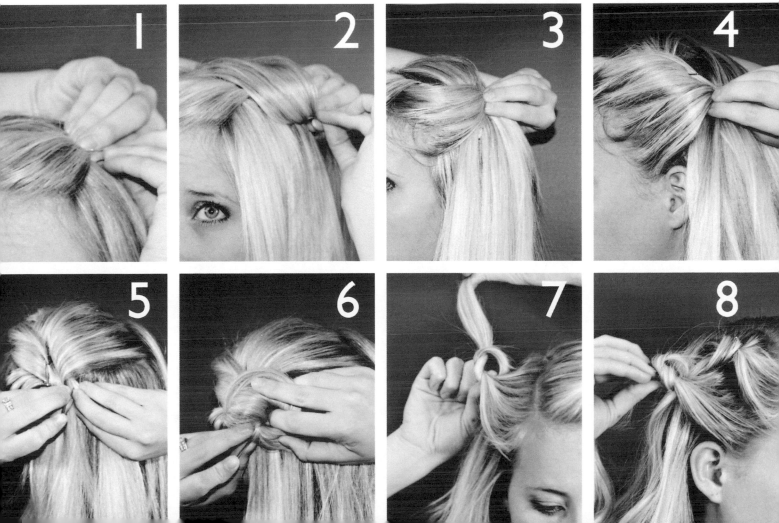

Twisties

1. Starting at the part, roll hair backwards
2. Continue rolling hair
3. Secure with bobby pin near top of ear
4. Take top section of hair from other side of head
5. Twist until it meets up with first bobby pin and secure with bobby pin
6. Take bottom section of hair and twist
7. Secure with bobby pin
8. Place flower over bobby pins

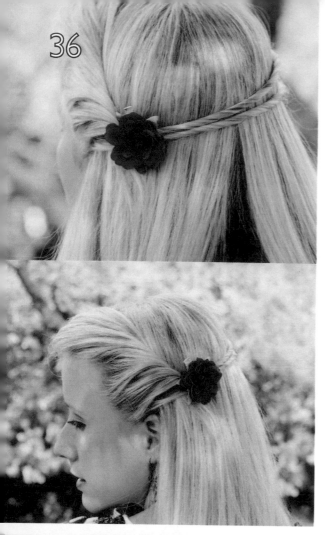

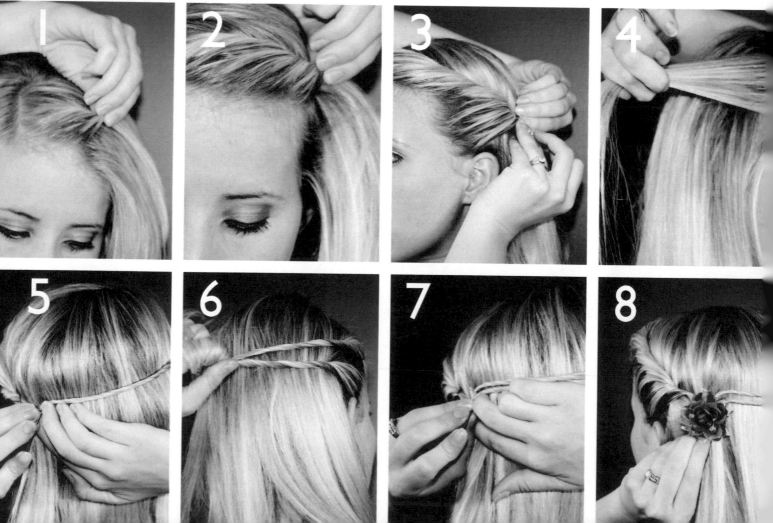

Waterfall Double Braids

1. French braid front section of hair
2. On second braid, drop top section through middle and start waterfall braid
   Note: Refer to waterfall braid tutorial
3. Waterfall braid all the way back and finish with regular braid
4. Secure with clear elastic
5. Start a regular french braid from the front using the pieces that fell from waterfall braid
6. Continue braiding back and secure with clear elastic
7. Put your hair up into a ponytail and undo clear elastics
8. For more formal look, pull hair back into fancy half-up
   Note: Once hair is secure, undo clear elastics and curl ends

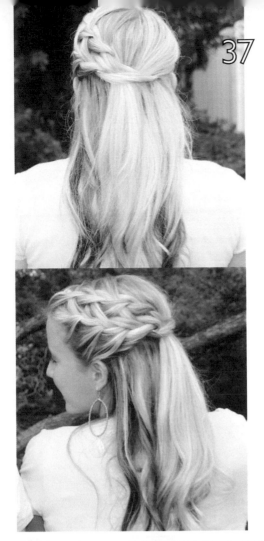

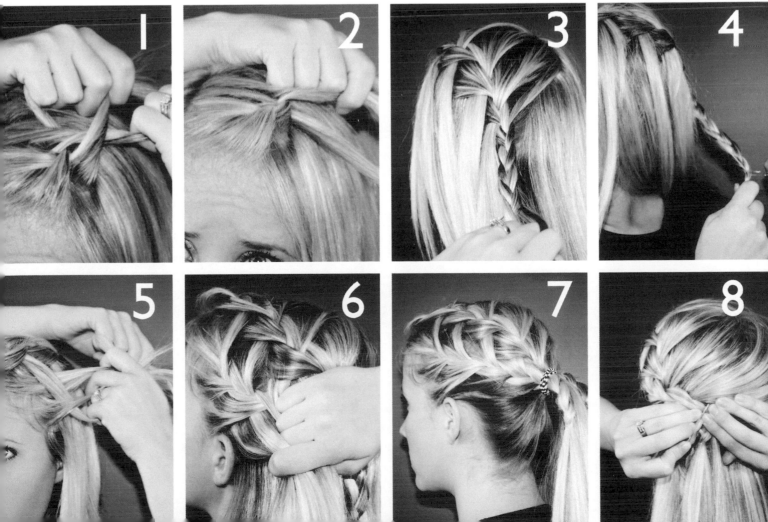

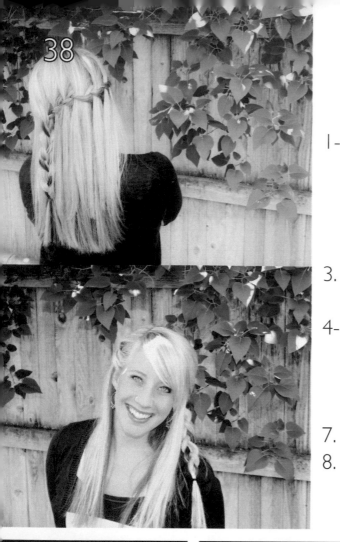

Waterfall Braid

Note: Start waterfall braid on thinner side. If this tutorial is confusing please refer to the video tutorial on my website

1-2. Begin with regular french braid. 3 strands. Bottom section over middle. Top section over middle. Add hair to bottom section take it over middle. Add hair to top section like normal. Take section over middle and drop section

3. Replace middle section with chunk of hair directly next to section that was just dropped

4-6. Keep braiding as if middle section had never been replaced. Add hair to bottom section and take it over the middle. Add hair to top section and drop it through the middle. Repeat

7. Take front section of hair and fold it over braid

8. Secure with bobby pins or continue braiding down tail securing with clear elastic

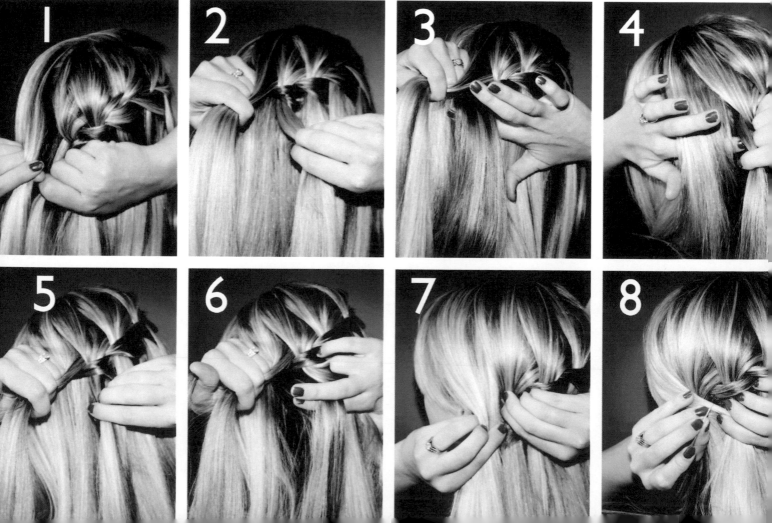

Waterfall Twist

1. Split hair into three sections
2. Take top section and drop it through the middle of the bottom two sections
3. Take bottom section and twist over top section
4. Add a new section of hair from the top
5. Drop that new section through middle
6. Take bottom section and twist over top section. Repeat steps 4-6.
7. Tie off twists with clear elastic

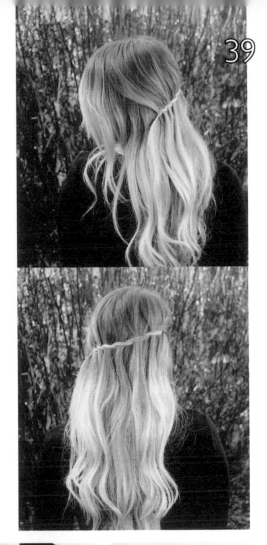

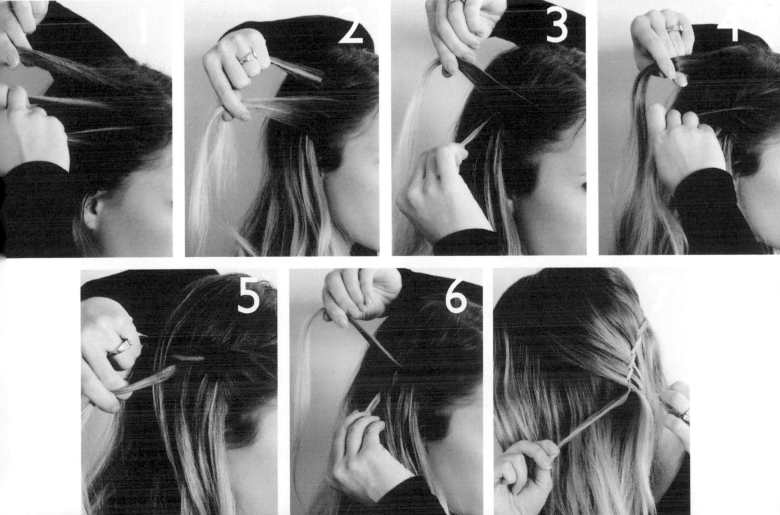

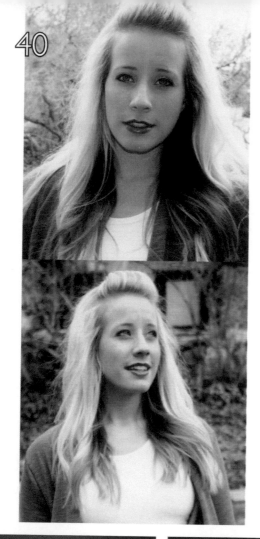

Wavy Poof

1-2. Pull bangs back with hand
3. While holding bangs, push them forward to create volume
4-5. Horizontally secure with bobby pins, one on each side
6. Hair spray
7. Rat
8. Push hair up with hands while hairspraying

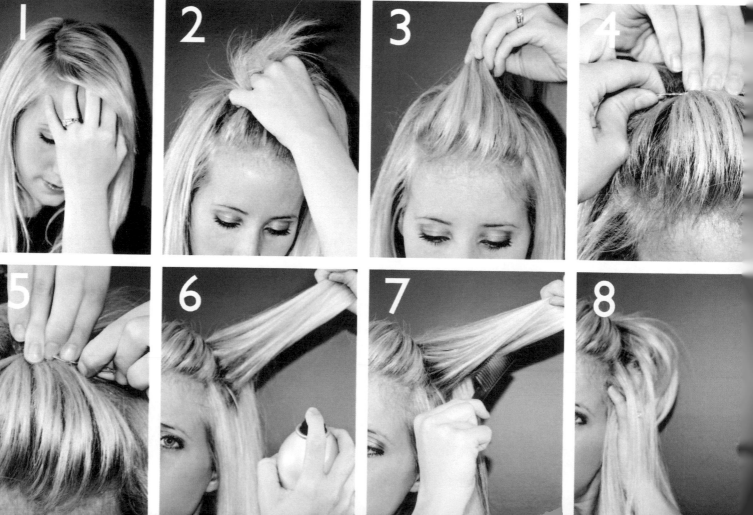

Wedding Bun

1. Pull front two sections back
2. Fold sections over each other and secure with bobby pin
3-4. Repeat steps 1-2

    Note: When finished pinning, fix any bubbles and loosen hair around crown

5-6. Take tail and twist around into bun
7-8. Bobby pin bun onto head

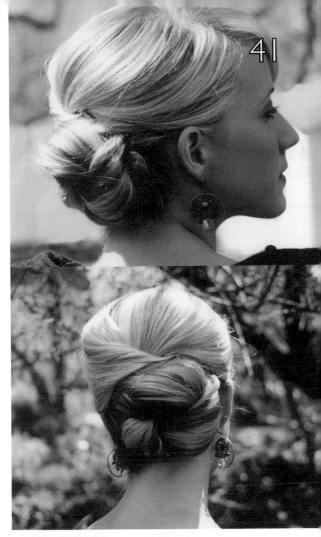

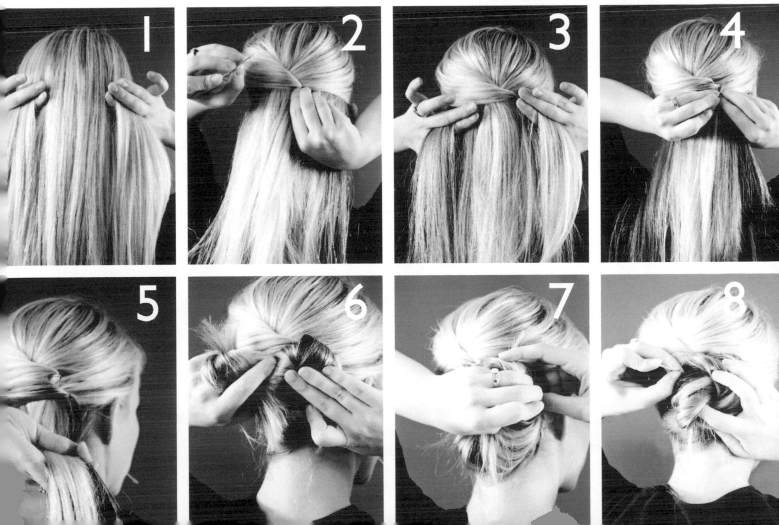